Boy or Girl?

50 Fun Ways to Find Out

Boy or Girl?

50 Fun Ways to Find Out

———— ❤ ————

Shelly Lavigne

Illustrated by
Penny Carter

A Dell Trade Paperback

Art Direction: **David Kaestle, Inc.**
Design & Production: **David Vogler**

Thanks to Fred Tunks and to all the people who
contributed their old wives' tales.

A DELL TRADE PAPERBACK

Published by Dell Publishing
a division of Bantam Doubleday Dell Publishing Group, Inc.
1540 Broadway
New York, New York 10036

ISBN: 0-440-50459-7

Printed in the United States of America

Published simultaneously in Canada

July 1992

30 29 28 27 26

Contents

To Brooke

Introduction

After I discovered I was pregnant with my first child, I was always asked: "What do you think it will be, a boy or a girl?" I became curious and started collecting old wives' tales that predict whether you're going to have a boy or a girl baby.

All you need to do is take out a piece of paper and number it 1 through 50, making two columns (one for *boy,* one for *girl*). As you take the "tests," record your results and total your score.

And there you are, all the folklore evidence you need to tell your friends whether you're going to have a baby boy or a baby girl!

CHAPTER ONE

Mom's Body

Giving birth to either a girl or a boy
is an event almost beyond imagination.
Each of us is a miracle. But we still have that
overwhelming curiosity about which sex is on
the way. This first chapter tells what's
happening to your body from
head to toe.

———— ❤ ————

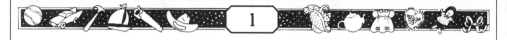

Mirror, Mirror on the Wall...

This old German tale checks not whether you are the fairest mother of all, but what your eyes say. Stare into the mirror for at least one minute, but not more than three.

Mom, do your eyes dilate?
If yes, a boy.

They don't? A girl.

❏ *Boy*

❏ *Girl*

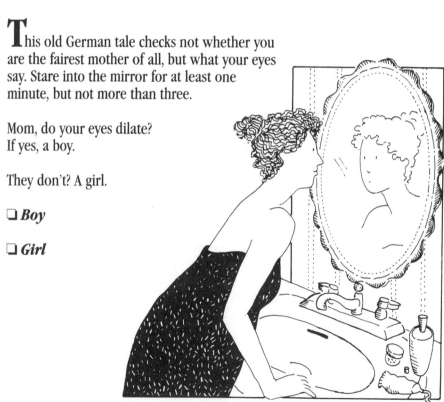

Eye Can Tell

Pull your lower eyelids down and look at the whites of your eyes. Do you see a broken blood vessel in the shape of a "V"?

If that "V" is in the lower half of your right eye, count on a boy.

❏ *Boy*

There's a girl coming if the "V"-shaped broken blood vessel is in your left eye.

❏ *Girl*

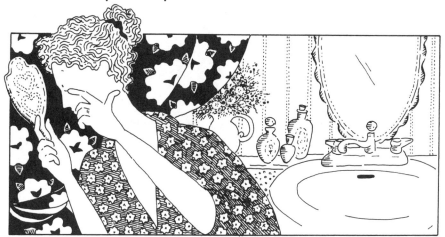

What Your Hair Reveals

Stay at the mirror, Mom, and comb your hair for a bit.

Is your hair getting thinner and stringier with each day of pregnancy? It is if you are pregnant with a girl child. Swedish folklore says so.

Or is your hair becoming more shiny and full-bodied? If so, the Swedes say it's a boy.

❏ *Boy*

❏ *Girl*

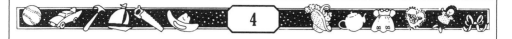

From Hair to There

While we're on the subject of hair, take a look at the hair on your legs.

If your leg hair is growing faster now, a boy is on the way. If your hair growth, legwise, is the same as before your pregnancy, you should be getting ready for a girl.

❏ *Boy*   ❏ *Girl*

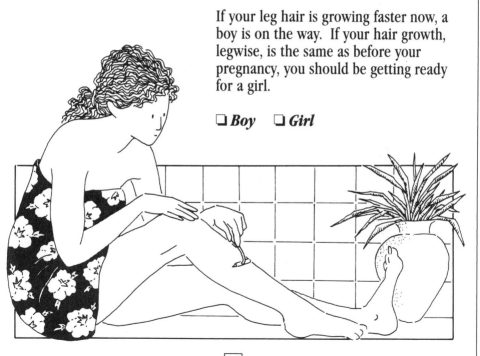

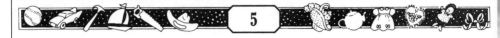

Another Leg Tale

French tale tellers look to Mom's legs for their clue. It's true that legs can put on weight during pregnancy.

Are your legs beginning to resemble "tree trunks"? A sure sign of a boy.

If your legs are just as trim as they were before you became pregnant, look for a girl at delivery time.

❏ *Boy*   ❏ *Girl*

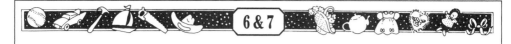

No Applause, Please

Mom, look closely at your hands. Are they rough or smooth? (And what do you think the sex indications would naturally be?)

You're right! A girl goes with smooth hands. That means a boy will be born to one with rough hands.   ❏ *Boy*   ❏ *Girl*

One More for the Hands

Mom, have your fingernails grown faster and stronger during pregnancy?

If yes, score another one in the *boy* column. And, Mom, if your nails haven't changed, check *girl.*

❏ *Boy*   ❏ *Girl*

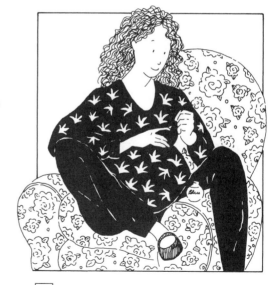

Back-end Blues

This time, Mom, check the weight gain on your backside.

Do you notice any weight gain back there? No? Congratulations, a boy is on the way.

But on the other hand, if there is more of you back there, think pink. A girl is right around the corner.

❏ *Boy*

❏ *Girl*

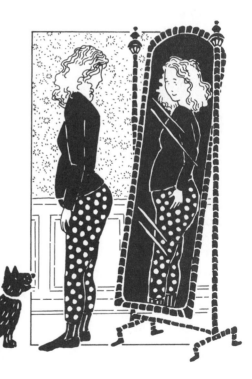

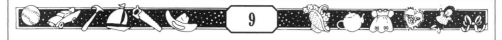

It Figures

Mom, it's time to bite the bullet and look at what's happening to your waistline.

Is that midsection pretty much straight up and down, or is it bulging? (This question, mind you, is appropriate after seven months or so of pregnancy.)

Mom, you are growing a boy inside if you can still see your waistline.

"What waistline?" you say. Bulging sides go along with a girl.

❑ *Boy* ❑ *Girl*

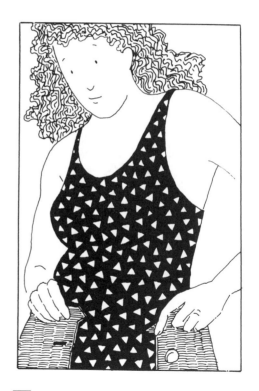

15

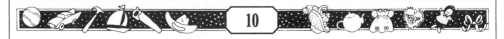
Facing the Facts

Time to check your face weight. Are you more ample about the face since pregnancy became a fact of life? Italians say that's what comes with having a girl. Still got your slender profile? It's a boy.

❏ *Boy*   ❏ *Girl*

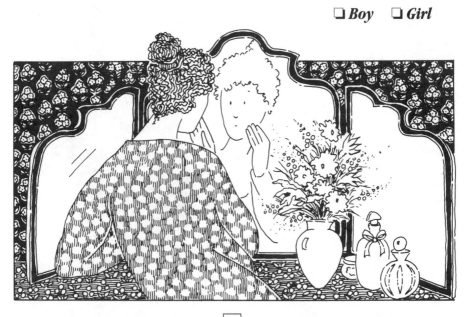

CHAPTER TWO

Clues for Mom

There are so many changes for Mom to
get used to, including feelings that you
probably haven't felt before. However strange
they may be, these feelings are part of
bringing a new life into the world. According to
folklore from around the world, what
Mom feels (or doesn't feel) can foretell
the coming of a boy or a girl.

❤

Getting Cold Feet?

Mom, are you bugged by your feet being colder than they were before your pregnancy?

No, you say? Your feet feel just about the same? Another score for a girl.

Mark one for a boy if your feet are often a bit chillier than before.

❏ *Boy*

❏ *Girl*

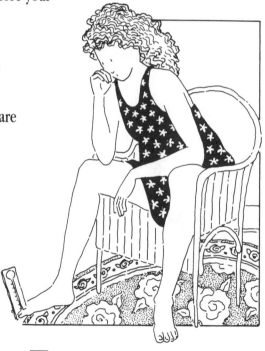

A Sense of Direction

Mom, a very old New England wives' tale says if you are sleeping in a bed with your head to the north, you'll have a boy.

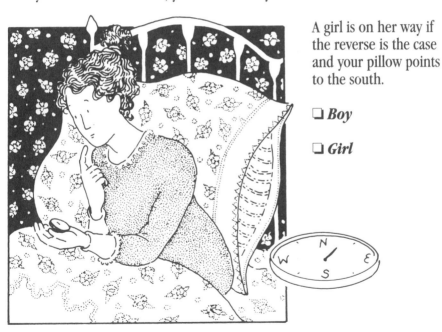

A girl is on her way if the reverse is the case and your pillow points to the south.

❏ *Boy*

❏ *Girl*

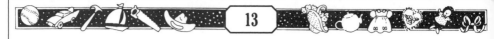

Call the Plumber

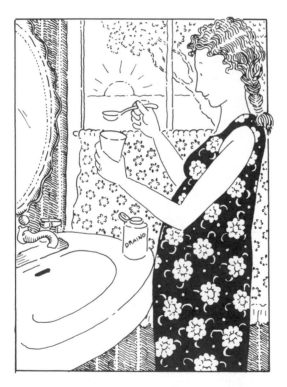

For this familiar American test, add one tablespoon of crystal Drano to a small amount of your first-of-the-morning urine, and wait a bit to see what happens.

Is the mixture turning a bluish yellow color? That signals a boy.

If it turns greenish brown, count on a baby girl.

❏ *Boy*

❏ *Girl*

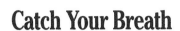

Catch Your Breath

Have you noticed breathing is more difficult since your pregnancy? A boy is on the way when you experience shortness of breath.

No problem? You're breathing free and easy? It's a girl.

❏ *Boy*

❏ *Girl*

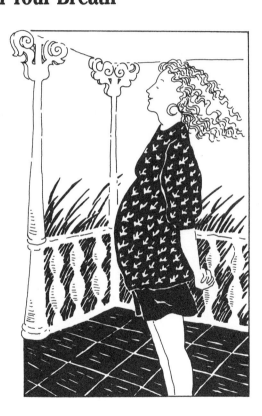

To the Heart of the Matter

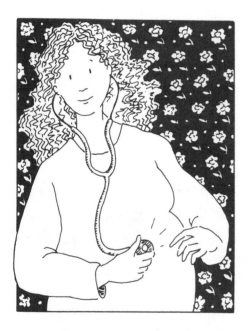

Mom, it's important for you to have a good doctor to ease you through your pregnancy. The next time you see your doc, take this quick sex test by asking for a check of your baby's heartbeat.

A rate of 139 or below indicates that it's a boy's heart that's beating.

If the reading is 140 or above, it's a girl's heart that will power a new life.

❏ *Boy*

❏ *Girl*

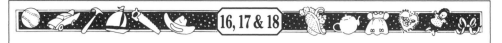

Sleepy Sylvia or Alert Albert?

Germans say that a girl will make you want to sleep more than you did before. But a boy won't make you so sleepy.

❏ *Boy*   ❏ *Girl*

Taking Sides

A girl is favored if you sleep on your right side. If your left side is your usual choice, it's a boy.

❏ *Boy*   ❏ *Girl*

Nocturnal Nonsense

Do you dream more often of having a boy or a girl?

❏ *Boy*   ❏ *Girl*

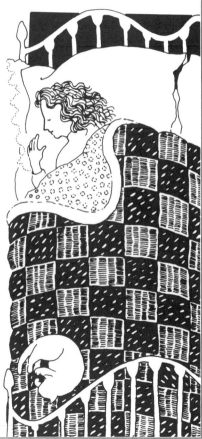

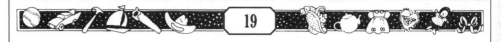
It's Better to Throw up Your Hands

Dad will say it's only natural for you to have morning sickness. Frequent nausea, he's heard for years, goes with being in a family way.

But according to the greater authority of old wives' tales, you are more likely to have morning sickness when a girl is in your tummy.

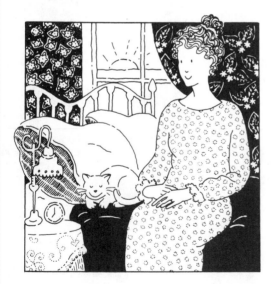

A boy, it is said, waits until he's born to upset you!

❑ *Boy*

❑ *Girl*

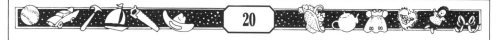

Due for an Overhaul?

Overall, do you feel well or not so well during your pregnancy?

Let's not question the wisdom or logic of this folklore, but it is said that bearing a son is the more comfortable way to go.

Having a daughter, it is said, makes for a more troublesome pregnancy.

❏ *Boy*

❏ *Girl*

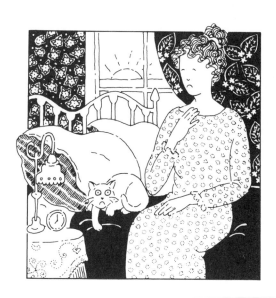

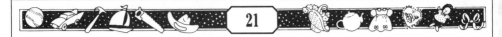

Grandma's Influence Is a Gray Area

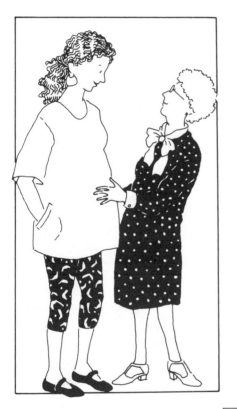

Does your mom–the child's maternal grandmother–have gray hair or is it colored? It doesn't really matter whether the gray or color is natural or dyed.

If Grandma has gray hair, a boy will be born.

If her hair is another color, a girl is headed for her coming-out party.

❑ *Boy*

❑ *Girl*

CHAPTER THREE

A Matter of Taste

Of course, Mom's changing food likes and dislikes can reveal all sorts of things about the sex of the Little One.

———❤———

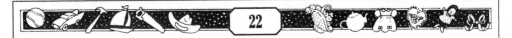

What's Cookin'?

Perhaps Dad and relatives and friends have noticed that you are busier than ever in the kitchen. Are you baking chocolate chip cookies when the jar is already overflowing? Or does a simple dinner turn out to be a feast of hors d'oeuvres, fancy salad, veggies of all colors, a succulent roast, and a pecan pie, which you've never baked before?

That hyper kitchen activity is happening
because there's a boy growing in your tummy.   ❏ *Boy*

Is the kitchen as dull a place as ever?
The score's in the *girl* box then.   ❏ *Girl*

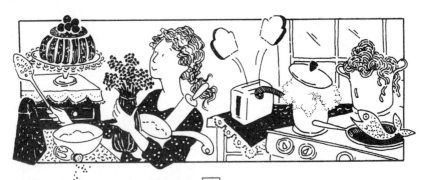

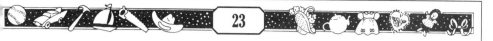
Sweet or Sour?

Fathers know that pregnancy can give you strange and overwhelming cravings for certain foods.

In Iowa, they ask if it's pickles or ice cream that you like so much. Sour pickles get the *boy* score.

A sweet girl goes with a taste for ice cream.

❏ *Boy*

❏ *Girl*

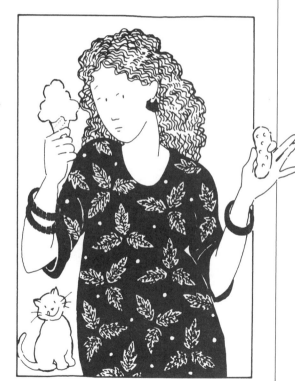

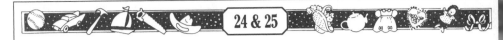

Don't Be a Heel

In Italy, bread is the key to this test. Now that you are pregnant, do you find yourself refusing the heel of a loaf of bread? If so, you're bearing a girl. If, on the other hand, you actually prefer the heel, score one more point for a boy.

❏ *Boy* ❏ *Girl*

Serious About Citrus

Mom, do you get up in the morning with the feeling that you must have a glass of orange juice? If so, a girl is what's growing.

If orange juice isn't on your mind every day, then count on a boy.

❏ *Boy* ❏ *Girl*

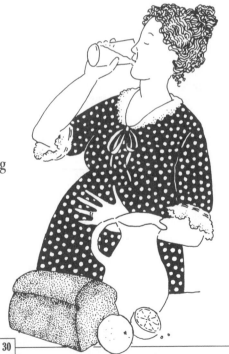

CHAPTER FOUR

Ask the Baby

Baby isn't talking, but she or he
certainly is communicating as Mom's delightful
wonder gets heavier and heavier and
more and more active.

Folklore around the world says
Baby's womb-bound movements provide
plenty of boy or girl hints.

———— ❤ ————

High or Low?

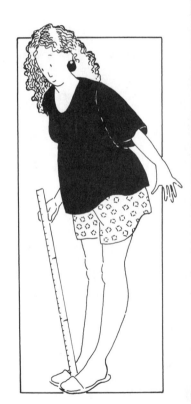

You probably already know whether you are carrying your baby high or low.

According to this old wives' tale, there's a message in your baby's position.

A high baby is a girl, or so it is recorded in the realm of folklore.

A low baby? You've got it...a boy.

❏ *Boy*

❏ *Girl*

The Shape of Things

Mom, take another look at that buldge that's getting bigger and bigger.

What does your stomach resemble, shapewise? Without stretching your imagination too far, does the pregnant part resemble a watermelon?

A sweet girl is the indication. More like a basketball? A sporty boy, naturally.

❏ *Boy*

❏ *Girl*

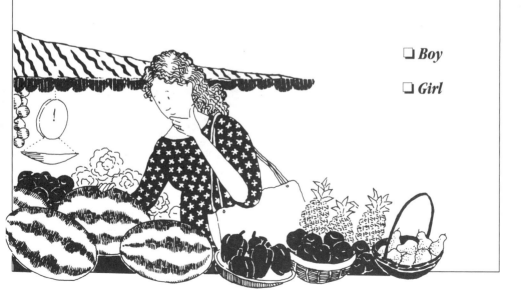

Getting a Kick Out of All This

Mom, you certainly are getting
a boot out of something. The little
one in there is becoming more
and more impatient.

Where do you get kicked
most often by your
little bundle? It's
been said that a boy
prefers the ribs.

The lower stomach is likely
to be the choice of a girl.

❏ *Boy*

❏ *Girl*

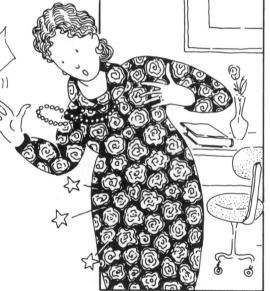

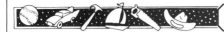 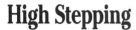

High Stepping

Do those tiny feet go flying to your left most frequently...or to the right? In this Norwegian wives' tale boys have an affinity for the right. Girls tend to kick to the left.

❏ *Boy*   ❏ *Girl*

Right Again

Mom, does the baby lie most frequently on the right or left side of your tummy? A boy will lie more often toward your left side. A girl tends to lie on the right.

❏ *Boy*   ❏ *Girl*

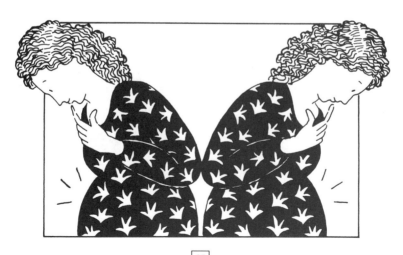

Let's Dance

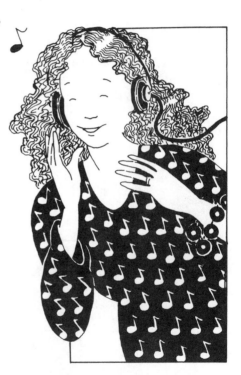

We can blame this one on a wives' tale that originated centuries ago in Vienna.

Supposedly, baby girls "dance" when they hear music.

Baby boys keep still and just listen.

❏ *Boy*

❏ *Girl*

CHAPTER FIVE

Just for Dad

While all the attention is being focused
on Mom, we need to remember that
Dad has a part in all this, too!

Here are some tests—as authentic as any of
the others—just for him.

———— ❤ ————

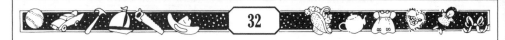

Something to Smile About

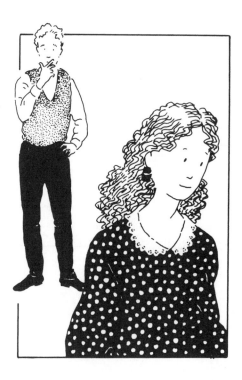

Do you see Mom smiling more since she got pregnant?

An affirmative answer means you've got a boy on the way.

If there are no more smiles or even fewer than before, folklore declares that attitude is brought on by a girl.

❏ *Boy*

❏ *Girl*

Uptight or Cool

Dad, there are many changes that come into your life when Mom gets pregnant. If you are more nervous now, expect a girl. A boy in the hopper will make you feel more relaxed.

❏ *Boy*   ❏ *Girl*

Handyman

A lot of household projects come packed in the pregnancy package. If you're getting more projects done around the house, there's a new son in your future. Dad, you're not lazy, but if you're really not doing any more than you did before, there's a new daughter in the making.

❏ *Boy*   ❏ *Girl*

How Much Weight Does Dad Carry?

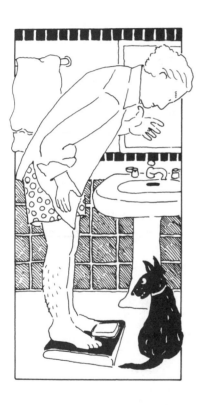

Sometimes fathers gain weight, too, with pregnancy. Nothing new in that. But maybe you don't know what it means when you get heavier as Mom's pregnancy advances. It means a boy is on the way.

If that's not the case and you are as trim as ever, or at least you're not putting on anything extra, you're looking ahead to the birth of a girl.

❏ *Boy*

❏ *Girl*

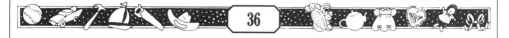

Wish Upon a Bone

Here's a test that calls for Mom and Dad to pull apart a dried turkey wishbone. No wishing this time; just see who gets the bigger piece.

Mom, is your part of the bone the bigger? Then you'll have a daughter, for sure.

Dad, did you win the pull? A son, of course.

❏ *Boy*   ❏ *Girl*

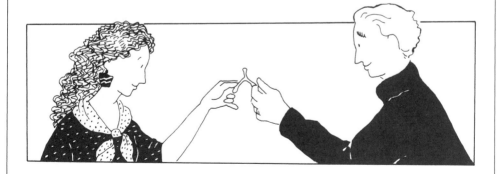

On Pins and Needles

Thread a needle and stick it into the eraser head of a pencil. Use the thread to dangle the pencil over Mom's wrist, then wait for the pencil to start moving.

If the pencil swings from side to side across Mom's wrist, there's a boy in Mom's future.

If the pencil swings parallel to Mom's arm and wrist, that's in keeping with the coming of a girl.

❏ *Boy*

❏ *Girl*

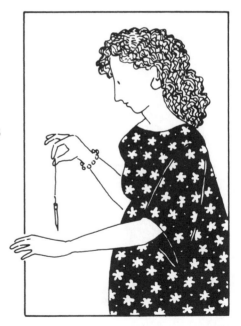

CHAPTER SIX

Mom Draws a Crowd

Most of all, Moms look forward to
celebrating the coming event with friends
at a shower or some other group activity.
This chapter is specifically for the
involvement of many. Have fun as your family
and friends go with you through these
boy/girl tales from many lands.

❤

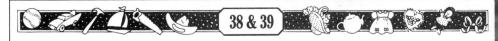

Hanky Panky

With the group as spectators, put a facial tissue flat on a table and ask Mom to pick it up. If she grabs the edge of the tissue, she will have a girl. If she grabs one of the four corners, she will have a boy.

❏ *Boy*　❏ *Girl*

Coffee, Tea, or...?

While you are all there at the table, offer Mom a cup of coffee and watch how she picks it up. If you see her pick it up by the handle, you can bet her child is a boy. But if, instead, Mom keeps her hands warm by holding the cup by its sides, mark the *girl* box.

❏ *Boy*　❏ *Girl*

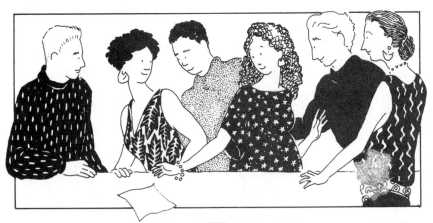

A Corny Surprise

A Romanian old wives' tale says to sneak up behind Mom and sprinkle a bit of cornmeal in her hair. Then hope she doesn't shake it out when she asks, "Why did you do that?"

Respond by asking Mom to touch her mouth or her nose.

Did she touch her mouth? It was the thing for her to do because she's pregnant with a girl baby.

Or did Mom touch her nose? You'd expect that to happen with a boy hiding in there.

❏ *Boy*

❏ *Girl*

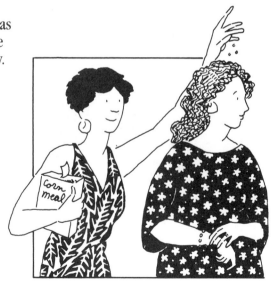

Pillow Talk

Put two pillows on the floor. Ask Mom to look the other way, then place a fork under one pillow and a spoon under the other.

Now get Mom's attention again and ask her to sit on one of the pillows.

If Mom sits on the pillow with the fork, she'll have a girl.

If she sits on the pillow with the spoon, Mom is telling you there's a boy on the way.

❑ *Boy*   ❑ *Girl*

Ring Around Rosey

While Mom's still there on the floor, ask her to give you her wedding ring. Then ask her to lie on the floor on her back.

Tie a string to Mom's wedding ring and hold the string so that the ring hangs three inches from Mom's stomach. Hold the string still.

When the ring swings, does it swing for a boy—hip to hip?

Or does it swing for a girl—the opposite way, up and down the stomach?

❏ *Boy*

❏ *Girl*

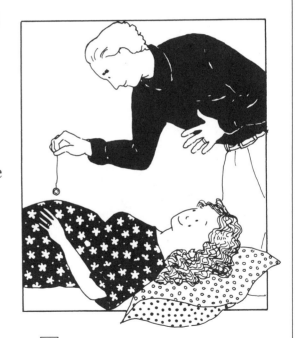

Time to Get Up

Tell Mom it's okay for her to get up now. Watch very closely as she gets up or you'll miss the tell-all of this one.

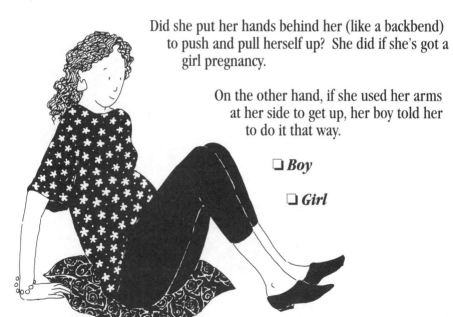

Did she put her hands behind her (like a backbend) to push and pull herself up? She did if she's got a girl pregnancy.

On the other hand, if she used her arms at her side to get up, her boy told her to do it that way.

❏ *Boy*

❏ *Girl*

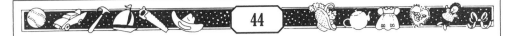

Neck and Neck

Take this clue from the Italians and ask Mom to pull her hair up from the back of her neck.

If you see new hair growth that forms a point or a "V," she's having a boy.

If you see new hair growing straight across her neck, it's because of the presence of a girl.

❏ *Boy*

❏ *Girl*

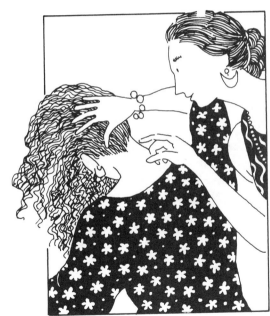

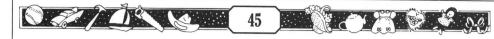

A Show of Hands

Ask Mom to show you her hands. How does she hold them out?

If she holds them out with her palms facing up, she did it the girl way.

Or did she do it the boy way–with palms facing down?

❏ *Boy*

❏ *Girl*

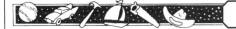

Unlock the Answer

Place a key in the palm of your hand and ask Mom to pick it up.

How does Mom grab it?

By the "teeth"? That's what Mom's girl will have her do.

Or by the key base? It's the boy in Mom that did it.

❏ *Boy*

❏ *Girl*

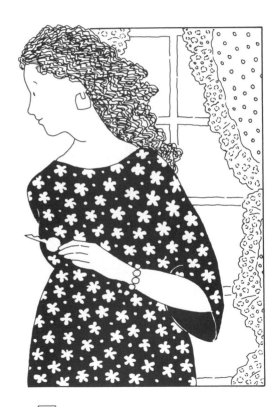

51

Itching for More

Test this bit of Romanian folklore by sneaking up behind Mom and sprinkling a bit of salt in her hair. It's more entertaining for the group if you can do it without Mom noticing. In about five or ten minutes look to see if Mom begins scratching her lips or nose.

If you see her go for her nose, she will have a boy.

If she scratches her lips, she's itching for a girl.

❏ *Boy*　　❏ *Girl*

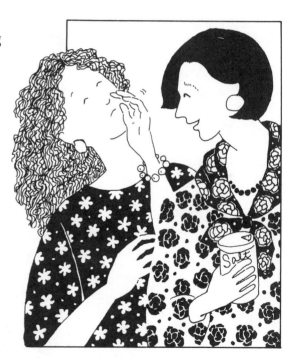

Wrap It Up

When it's time for Mom to open her gifts, test this old wives' tale. If she opens them neatly and saves the bows, you're looking at a girl in her future. If that's not the case, and Mom rips open the paper and tosses the bows, her gift will be a boy.

❏ *Boy*   ❏ *Girl*

Color Baby Beautiful

As Mom opens her gifts, what color baby clothing does she receive more of? The answer is green if Mom is expecting a boy. The answer is yellow if Mom has a girl to present.

❏ *Boy*

❏ *Girl*

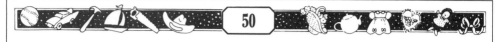

The Hand Off

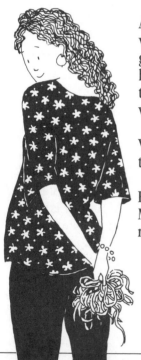

Now that Mom is gushing with joy over all the beautiful gifts she has received, here's a girl/boy test that gets everyone involved.

Ask Mom for her engagement or wedding ring and wrap all the ribbons around it in a ball. Have all the guests stand in a circle with Mom in the center. Then have the guests pass the ball of ribbon from one to the other behind their back, unraveling the ribbon with each passing.

Watch carefully as the ring reappears! Is the ring in the receiving person's left or right hand?

Folklore has it that if the ring is in the right hand, Mom will have a girl. There's a boy on the way if the ring landed in the left hand.

❏ *Boy*   ❏ *Girl*

CHAPTER SEVEN

An Oriental Orientation

It's important to know, as you use the following chart, that its structure is based on the month of the baby's conception, not on the month of the baby's birth.

The mother's age, from 18 to 45, is on the top line, with the months of conception at the left. Just match your age on the horizontal axis to the month of your baby's conception on the vertical axis and there you have it, your newfound knowledge of whether to expect a boy (M) or a girl (F).

❤

CHINESE CONCEPTION

Woman's Conceiving Age

Month of Conception	18	19	20	21	22	23	24	25	26	27	28	29
January	F	M	F	M	F	M	M	F	M	F	M	F
February	M	F	M	F	M	M	F	M	F	M	F	M
March	F	M	F	F	M	F	M	M	M	F	M	F
April	M	F	M	F	F	M	M	F	F	M	F	F
May	M	F	M	F	M	M	F	F	F	F	F	M
June	M	M	M	F	F	F	M	M	M	F	F	M
July	M	M	M	F	F	M	M	F	F	M	M	M
August	M	M	M	F	M	F	F	M	M	M	M	M
September	M	M	M	F	F	M	F	M	F	M	M	M
October	M	M	F	F	F	M	F	M	F	M	M	F
November	M	F	M	F	F	M	F	M	F	F	F	F
December	M	F	M	F	F	F	F	M	F	M	F	F

CHART

Just match your age with the month of baby's conception...

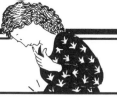

Woman's Conceiving Age

30	31	32	33	34	35	36	37	38	39	40	41	42	43	44	45
M	M	M	F	M	M	F	M	F	M	F	M	F	M	M	F
F	F	F	M	F	M	M	F	M	F	M	F	M	F	M	M
F	M	M	M	M	F	M	M	F	M	F	M	F	M	F	M
F	F	F	M	F	M	F	M	M	M	M	F	M	F	M	F
F	F	F	F	F	F	M	F	M	M	F	M	F	M	M	F
F	F	F	F	F	F	F	M	F	F	M	F	M	F	M	F
F	F	F	F	F	F	F	F	M	F	M	M	F	M	F	M
F	F	F	M	F	M	F	M	F	M	F	M	M	F	M	F
F	F	F	F	F	F	M	F	M	F	M	F	M	M	F	M
F	F	F	F	F	F	M	M	F	M	F	M	F	M	M	F
M	F	F	F	M	M	M	F	M	F	M	F	M	M	F	M
M	M	M	M	M	M	M	M	F	F	F	M	F	M	F	M

Of course, if you are reading this book before you conceive, you can use this chart to try to plan the sex of your baby-to-be.

This chart, according to Chinese history, was created by a scientist in the thirteenth century and then buried in a royal tomb near Beijing. The original chart is now kept in the Institute of Science of Beijing. The chart has a reputation in China for being 99% accurate, having been proven, it is said, by millions of mothers.

This claim of accuracy is supported to a great extent here in the United States. For example, two OBGYNs at the Aspen Medical Center have been checking the chart's boy/girl forecasting abilities for some time, and the accuracy rate has been running about 85%. And the chart has generated a great deal of interest among the patrons of a Minnesota beauty salon by showing an accuracy rate of 90%.

Which is right?

❏ The results of your series of tests?

❏ Or the wisdom of the Chinese?

❏ Maybe both!

CHAPTER EIGHT

It's Not Over till It's Over

By now you have taken dozens of tests in order to determine which sex to expect for your new baby. And you've checked this result with the wisdom of the ancient Chinese. But even though Baby already has been conceived, what follows is more folklore from here and there that says it's still not too late for Mom and Dad to have an influence on the sex of The One that's on the way. For instance...

———❤———

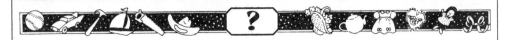

Pink or Blue?

It's still not too late to make a baby girl, according to one old wives' tale.

If you prefer a girl, just sleep with a pink ribbon under your pillow!

If you prefer a boy, place a blue ribbon under your pillow and your baby-boy wish will come true.

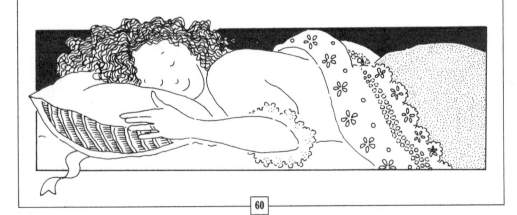

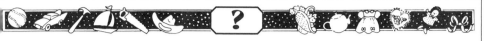

Shaking in His Boots

Dad's back in the picture for this one.

Let's say Dad puts sugar in his shoes as you are about to deliver. The more the better. You can bet he's got *his* bets on a girl.

Or when you start with your labor pains, is his first move to shake salt into his shoes? Well, we can guess he'd rather have a boy.

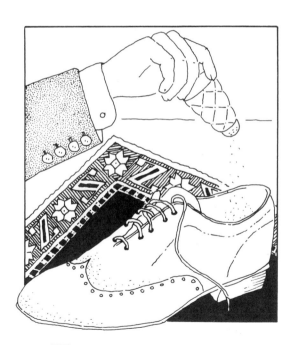

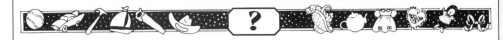

Into the Wild Blue Yonder

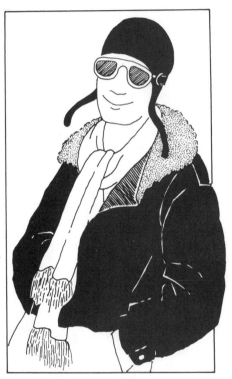

If a girl is the choice of heir, perhaps it's not too late, if Dad has a desire to take flying lessons…

Folklore has it that a girl will be born if Dad is a pilot.

If Dad says solid ground is fine for him, he'll have a boy to go fly a kite with.

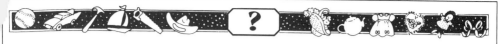

Onion and Garlic

Swedish folklore gives you, Mom, the power to influence the sex of your baby.

Your pregnancy will shift into male gear if you carry a garlic bud with you wherever you go.

What's it take for a shift to a female? You might have guessed. An onion must be your constant companion.

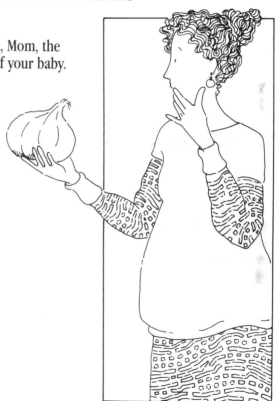

To My Baby from Mom

———❤———

Dear .... ,

   During the time I was expecting you, I had a lot of fun doing these little tests with your dad and our friends. According to the outcome, you were supposed to be a ....

   Lo and behold, you were a .... ! Of course, I would have loved you if you were a boy or a girl!

Lots of love,

Mom

P.S. Tuck this book away with your baby scrapbook, and think of me.